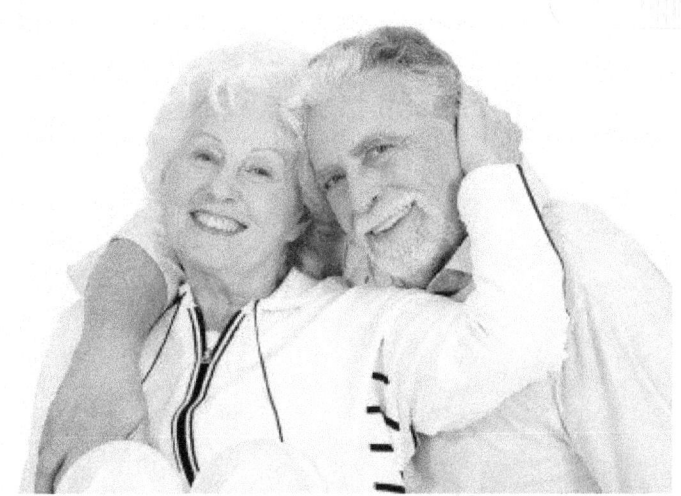

Photo by Ambro- freedigitalphotos.net

50 TIPS FOR FINDING ALZHEIMER'S GIFT IDEAS FOR THE HOLIDAYS (and other special events)

"I'm Out of Gift Ideas For My Alzheimer's Loved One What Can I Buy Them for Christmas?"

50 Suggestions from Penelope Mont,

Geriatric Consultant and

Recreation Therapist

Beaufort, South Carolina

2014

The following list of suggestions

can be modified to be

appropriate and enjoyed by

people in different levels of dementia.

1. <u>Homemade meals-</u>

    Finger foods with a touch of

    sweetness.

    Provide one serving at a time.

2. <u>Comfortable easy on/off clothes-</u>

This reduces frustration

and helps the caregiver.

(monogram)

3. <u>Fruit basket</u> –

   Include their favorites without pits and stems

   which might be eaten.

4. <u>Slippers/ velcro</u> -

   Must fit properly to prevent falls or slips-

   colors will help visibility-add name also.

5. <u>Large print books</u>-

   These can be on any level on their interest-

   don't be too childish.

6. <u>Old time music</u> -

   CD's or recordings from their era.

   These can be shared with others .

7. <u>Stuffed animal toys-</u>

>Musical, soft, collectible, large or small.

>(record your family's voices)

8. <u>Classic movies/nature tapes-</u>

>Farm, baby or pet animals

>plus funny old time TV shows.

9. <u>Baby dolls</u>—

>Clothes and doll cradles to bring back long ago memories. Holding brings pleasure.

10. <u>Old TV show's guessing games and matching stars-</u>

>Create or buy & try

>Other music games.

11. <u>Lap pad/tray for activities/eating-</u>

>For use in bed or chair.

>Puzzles can be kept on and finished later.

12. <u>Clock</u> – with day/date/ year –

    large size, not digital and

    place one in each room.

13. <u>Senior activity books-</u>

    Large print books,

    fun and colorful –

    a level for success but not childish.

14. <u>Lava lamp or moving fish tank lamp-</u>

    Fun to watch each day and is

    very calming-

    not breakable.

15. <u>Simple crafts</u> –

    Buy at dollar store and do together

    or with grandkids.

    Use as his gifts to others.

16. <u>Plan special outing/visit-</u>

Something to look forward to is always fun but don't forget the camera.

17. <u>Note pads, sticky notes</u> –

    Large colored crayons plus colored paper for special cards, etc.

18. <u>Lg. calendar-</u>

    Family or caregiver can write upcoming events, appointments and special dates.

19. <u>Make scrapbook-</u>

    or memory picture box with family, pets & activities from today and yesterday.

20. <u>Lg. wooden music box-</u>

    Bedtime music rituals add a Pleasant ending for the day.

21. <u>Rhythm band instruments with marching music</u> –

    Enough to share with his "band."

22. <u>Massages</u> –

    Find a service that will go

    to an Assisted Living

    home or to your house.

23. <u>Lap blanket with name on</u>-

    must be washable.

24. <u>Pet visits and trip to SPCA</u>-

    Help plan a trip out with the Activities Director.

    Volunteer your time/help.

25. <u>Electronic photo albums</u>-

    Revolving family pictures from

    today and also from years past.

26. <u>Microwavable neck pads-</u>

Hot or cold pads to reduce

stiffness and pain.

Kept by caregiver for his use.

27. <u>Bubble bath with calming</u>

<u>lavender scent</u> -

Kept by caregiver for

bath-time use.

28. <u>Play tea set, dishes, pots and pans, etc.</u>-

Pretend time helps with good memories and comfort feelings.

29. <u>Sm. recorder for reminders, family messages or music.</u>

Can be plastic to prevent breakage.

30. <u>Costume jewelry – for both men and ladies</u>.

(watches, bracelets, rings, etc.)

And special box.

31. <u>Grandchild's homemade gifts-</u>

    Everything from pictures to a bunch of Fall leaves in a vase.

32. <u>Chair mini foot peddle bike-</u>

    A fun way to exercise !!

33. <u>Christmas tree ornament</u>.

    Buy a kit to made together and add date. Give as gifts or use on his door.

34. <u>Towels with Lg. print name-</u>

    Decorated with favorite animals or sports.

35. <u>Picture books- WW II, Nam, Air force, Navy or Army-</u>

They will remember !

(add a flag to keep)

36. <u>Automatic pill dispenser-</u>
Filled and set for
two weeks at a time
with sound and light reminders.

37. <u>Bean bag toss floor game-</u>
A fun activity to play
when you visit
or have visitors.

38. <u>Simplified TV remote</u> –
keep frustration low and
keep control feelings intact.

39. <u>Books</u> ---
Trains, planes, cars, dogs,
cats, farm animals,
tools, etc.

(Large colorful pictures)

40. <u>Toy realistic plastic tool case-
    treasure box</u>.
    His own box to keep things in.

41. <u>Grandma's lemon cake-</u>
    Enough to share with friends and staff.

42. <u>Basket for tissues, TV guide,</u>
    plus <u>snacks , glasses, keys, etc.</u>
    One for each Holiday ☺

43. <u>Bulletin board for notes, pictures,</u>
    plus <u>cards and reminders</u>.
    Include Holiday decorations to add.

44. <u>Busy board with locks & keys-</u>
    Things stay in place and keeps
    hands busy with familiar tasks.

45. <u>'Sports' night-light and mug-</u>

Other themed night-lights also. One for room and bathroom.

46. <u>Gospel/church songs</u> –

    Old familiar songs are never forgotten

    and enjoyed by listening or singing.

47. <u>Safe return bracelet</u> –

    Purchase at most pharmacy's or medical stores.

    ID might be needed !!

48. <u>Family picture tree-</u>

    Hang on room wall

    with real branches

    for pictures and names.

49. <u>Outside window birdfeeder-</u>

    You can watch the birds but

    they cannot see you. Fun !

50. <u>Windowsill planter-</u>

Watch bulbs bloom – plant together and provide a small plastic watering can.

Thank you everyone!!

I love getting gifts and

seeing everyone happy ☺

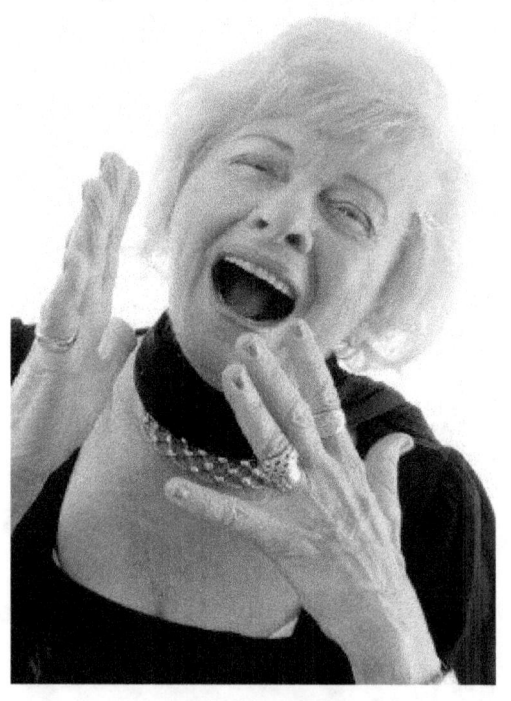

Photo by imagermajestic at FreeDigitalPhotos.net

Remember to keep the mail

coming, call me and please

visit me often!   (the best gifts).

****

NOW FOR A NEW ADDITION TO THIS

TIPS BOOK-   WE CAN'T FORGET THE

WONDERFUL CAREGIVERS !!

We all know how hard the Caregivers/ aides/ med techs/ Kitchen staff / housekeeping and Maintenance departments work. So let's keep them on our THANK YOU lists for their earned recognition. Since you will know each helper for your loved one best and what they might need and like, these are suggestions that you can change to fit each helper. These extra tips have helped me and used by me as an Activities Director for many Years. They have worked and have made a difference.

8 SUGGESTION/IDEAS/TIPS

1) Give a large dried fruit
   Basket assortment.
   Most other families give
   Cookies, cakes, candy, etc.
   All staff seem to get too
   much fattening treats at
   the holidays.
   Dried fruits look so pretty
   and can be left out in the
   break room without
   refrigeration. Good for
   all departments.

2) Gift cards to Wall Mart
   are so very welcomed.
   (Wall Mart has everything)
   Exact amounts can be
   changed for your 'special
   people' who serve your
   loved one with service
   beyond the call of duty.
   NOTE: some communities
   discourage money giving but

have a Caregiver Fund that you can contribute to.

3) Gas Cards- Everyone needs car gas to get to work. You could have a contest to guess the number of buttons in a jar. The closes guess gets a $30.00 gas card and the next closes gets a $20.00 card. WHAT FUN ☺

4) Set up a special massage day to relax and thank all Caregivers. Hire a friend who does massages and who will come to the Assisted living for 2 hours. (set up for staff breaks and shift changes)

5) Provide Holiday decorations

for Caregiver stations and break rooms. (do for several holidays throughout the year.)

6) Provide all materials for creating decorations for wheelchairs and walkers. The caregivers are very creative and most enjoy helping the residents to make their floor outstanding.

7) Donate holiday craft kits to the Activities Department. They usually have a fixed budget and welcome any special donations.

8) Provide a Subscription to the community for

<u>Oriental Trading</u> for fun and inexpensive gift ideas for any holiday throughout the year. Crafts are easy to make for all residents.

WWW.Orientaltrading.com

Giving and showing personal recognition and thanks is a very thoughtful and meaningful gift. Just your personal note in a card to that special helper is worth gold.

You receive that wonderful feeling that is the best part of giving at the Holidays.

BEST WISHES TO ALL

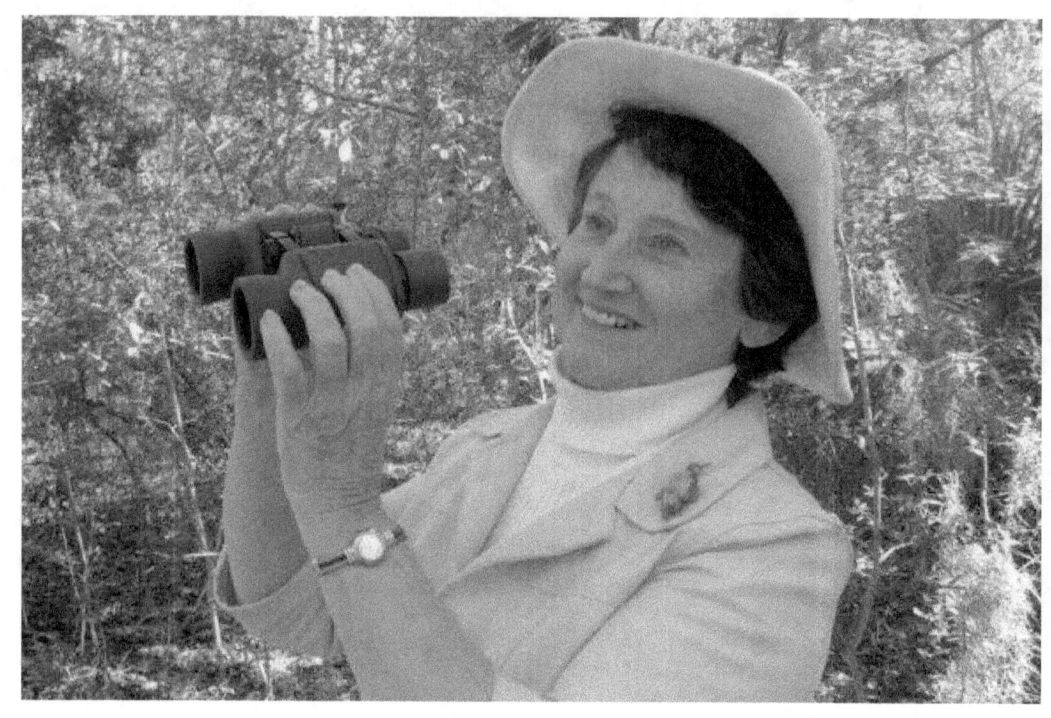

STILL LOOKING ?

IDEA- Give this list to your Children and Grandchildren.

Let them create ideas and make their own gifts with their own special touch.

Older children probably can create personal videos and photo slide shows.

Add music and watch for the smiles ☺

Kids can always bring their own personalities and fun to entertain the Grandparents in any situation.

How about putting on a little play or dance for the

whole Assisted Living home?

Your loved one can feel the joy and pride of having their family share with everyone. (idea- provide sodas since that is a rare treat.)

Holidays are fun for the memory loss population.

They live in the moment and are easy to please.

Watch your Holiday Stress and don't let it spill over onto your loved one.

It is a good idea to always check with their caregiver for gift ideas to fit the level needed.

Last year's successful gifts might not be appropriate this year.

Become a detective and discover what might work.

If it is not wanted at that moment, it might become a favorite in a month or two.

Note, they probably will not remember who gave the gift to them but will enjoy it anyway.

We all have to remember that there can be no new learned skills in advanced stages .

Keep projects and activities stimulating, fun and not too frustrating for them so that they can feel success.

Involve them in looking in gift catalogues, wrapping gifts and preparing food.

By being creative, we can find the "little child" inside our senior population.

Remember, the best part is

opening presents- soooo, wrap lots of little gifts to keep them busy and smiling.

Find more suggestion on-line.

Good luck and have fun.

HAPPY HOLIDAYS TO ALL

ABOUT THE AUTHOR

Penelope Mont's work experience includes: Special Ed Teacher; Geriatric Recreation therapy; Director of an Alzheimer's Day Center program; Director of Sales and

Marketing for an Assisted living/dementia community.

Penelope lives by the water in Beaufort, South Carolina with her big dog, Bart. She enjoys kayaking, shrimping, and especially visits from her two daughters and grandchildren.

She can be contacted via e-mail:

pmont@hargray.com

She would welcome any suggestions to add to this list.

Copyright 2011 & 2014

BARTSTER PUBLICATIONS

And PMSolutions LLC

Seabrook, SC 29940

www.ingramcontent.com/pod-product-compliance
Lightning Source LLC
Chambersburg PA
CBHW070734180526
45167CB00004B/1751